MARIE CURIE

The Pioneer of Radioactivity

Written by Justine Dutertre
In collaboration with Aurélie Le Floch
Translated by Rebecca Neal

History 50MINUTES.com

MARIE CURIE

KEY INFORMATION

- **Born:** 7 November 1867 in Warsaw, Congress Kingdom of Poland, Russian Empire (modern-day Poland).
- **Died:** 4 July 1934 in Passy, Haute-Savoie, France.
- **Main achievements:**
    - The discovery of radium and polonium (alongside her husband Pierre Curie, 1898).
    - Pioneering work on radioactivity, which she was the first person to define.
- **Impact:**
    - The development of innovative cancer treatments.
    - Awarded the Nobel Prize in Physics in 1903 and the Nobel Prize in Chemistry in 1911.

INTRODUCTION

Marie Curie broke new ground in scientific research in the late 19th and early 20th centuries: her work on radioactivity disproved the centuries-old belief that matter is indivisible and unchangeable, and her discovery of the radioactive elements radium and polonium paved the way for revolutionary new medical treatments.

Curie was fiercely ambitious and left her native Poland to study in France, where she lived in extreme poverty and had to make her way in a misogynistic, virtually impenetrable scientific world which rarely accepted women or gave their work the credit it deserved. However, her innate stubbornness and the challenges she weathered throughout her life gave her an extraordinary strength of character which allowed her to overcome these obstacles.

Pierre Curie (1859-1906) became her partner in life and work, and they experienced both great success and major challenges together. In addition to her international renown as a scientist, Curie has been held up as a pioneering feminist figure and a modern mother who was far ahead of her time, courageously returning to the laboratory shortly after giving birth to her two children. She fought for her ideals her entire life, and was responsible for significant advances not only in the field of medicine, but also in popular perceptions of women and their capabilities.

BIOGRAPHY

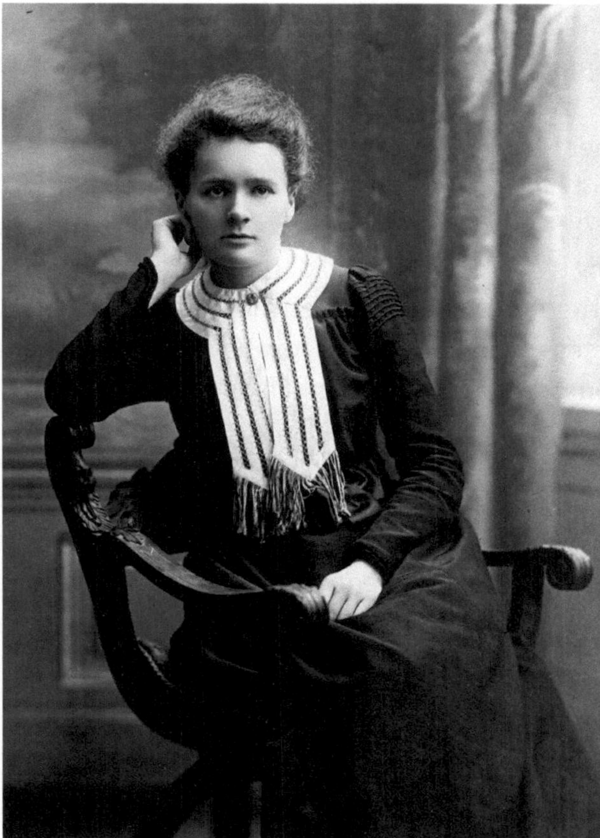

| Photograph of Marie Curie, c. 1903.

A HAPPY BUT TURBULENT CHILDHOOD

Marie Curie was born Maria Salomea Skłodowska in Warsaw on 7 November 1867, the youngest of five siblings. Her father Władysław Skłodowski (1832-1902) was a mathematics and physics teacher with a particularly keen interest in physics, and her mother Bronisława Skłodowska (died in 1878) also worked as a teacher before contracting tuberculosis. Her parents were loving but struggled to show it: her mother concealed her illness from her children and avoided physical contact with them as much as possible.

Maria was a precocious child: by the age of four, she could read perfectly, but her parents tried to hide more challenging books from her to preserve her innocence and prevent any harmful effects on her developing brain. She was irresistibly drawn to her father's test tubes and physics equipment, which were kept in a glass case in the family's living room, and would often sit and contemplate them.

In the space of just two years, Maria's mother died of tuberculosis and her sister Zofia died of typhus. She coped with her loss by throwing herself into her studies at the Flying University, a clandestine educational institution in Warsaw, where she focused in particular on mathematics.

EARLY ACADEMIC PROMISE

Later on, Maria worked as a governess for a family of wealthy farm owners while also secretly teaching a class of students in the countryside. She made a pact with her elder sister Bronisława; Bronisława would go to study in Paris while Maria and her father would work to support her, and later on Maria would join her in the French capital and embark on her own studies while Bronisława worked to support her. Consequently, Maria worked as a governess for three years, before returning to Warsaw to teach.

By 1891, Maria found her situation unbearable and left for Paris, where she assumed the French version of her first name, Marie, and enrolled in the science faculty at the Sorbonne. She was behind many of the other students and had to work hard to fill in the gaps in her knowledge. She moved in with Bronisława, who was now a gynaecologist, and her new husband Kazimierz Dłuski, a doctor, on the Rue d'Allemagne, but soon found this living situation suffocating as the couple both regularly received patients in their apartment. Marie subsequently moved into a sixth-floor maid's room without heating, electricity or running water; however, it was quiet and much closer to the university.

She worked tirelessly for three years, and during this period her life revolved entirely around her classes and revision. She lived a spartan existence: her meals often consisted of bread and butter and tea, and although she occasionally bought coal to heat her room, most of the time she slept in the cold and wore as many layers of clothes as possible to keep warm. Although she endured these difficult conditions uncomplainingly, on more than one occasion her brother-in-law found her unconscious from cold or hunger in her modest lodgings.

A BRILLIANT BUT REBELLIOUS STUDENT

Before long, Marie spoke perfect French, and continued to work as hard as ever. She eagerly followed the classes given by the physicists

Gabriel Lippmann (1845-1921) and Edmond Bouty (1846-1922) and the mathematicians Paul Painlevé (1863-1933) and Paul Appell (1855-1930), and her efforts soon paid off. In July 1893, she graduated top of her class with a physics degree, and was awarded a grant for high-achieving Polish students studying abroad. The following summer, she received a mathematics degree, this time graduating second in her class.

Marie joined Lippmann's team in France's leading physics laboratory, where she studied the magnetic properties of different types of steel. Although she found this work fascinating, she had a natural independent streak and wanted to carry out her own research. At a dinner, the Polish physicist Józef Wierusz-Kowalski (1866-1927), who was based at the University of Freiburg, introduced her to the 35-year-old Pierre Curie, who was an instructor at the School of Physics and Chemistry in Paris and shared her interest in the magnetic properties of metals. The instant physical, intellectual, emotional and spiritual attraction they felt developed into a close relationship, and the couple married on 26 July 1895. They went on to work together, and their shared goals and passion for physics and hard work made them an incredibly effective team.

In 1895 and 1896, Marie studied for the examination to teach mathematics to young girls, and although she graduated first in her class, she did not let this distract her from her ultimate goal of completing her doctoral thesis. On 12 September 1897, she gave birth to her first daughter, Irène, but she went back to work immediately afterwards, leaving the baby with a nurse most days so that she could focus on her research.

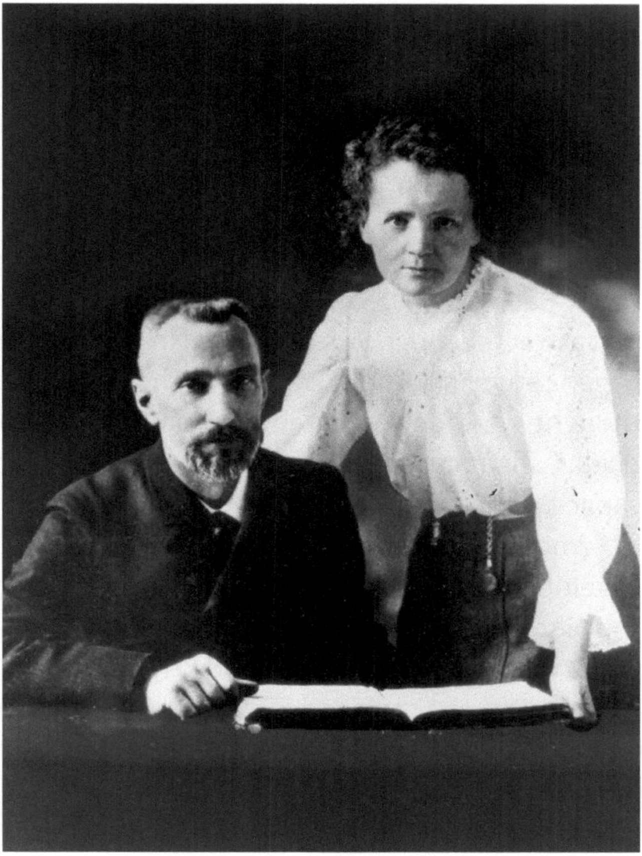

| Photograph of Pierre and Marie Curie, 1903.

DISCOVERING RADIUM

At this time, she was still looking for a subject for her thesis. X-rays, which had been discovered by the German physicist Wilhelm Röntgen (1845-1923) in 1895, had caused a major stir in the scientific world, but a similar type of ray discovered by Henri Becquerel (1852-1908) the following year had attracted much less attention. In 1897, Marie began studying these rays, which Becquerel thought were only emitted by uranium. In particular, she focused on quantifying their ionising capacity (meaning their ability to add charge to or remove charge from an atom) on the air, and developed a new system of measurement using the piezoelectric quartz electrometer (an instrument which can be used to study the radioactivity of different radioactive substances and the intensity of the radiation they emit) developed by Pierre Curie and his brother Jacques.

The Becquerel family

Henri Becquerel, who was born in Paris in 1852, was the grandson of the French physicist Antoine Becquerel (1788-1878), who was responsible for significant advances in research on electricity, its development and its applications. Henri's father, Edmond Becquerel (1820-1891), was also a French physicist and worked on spectrography. Henri discovered radioactivity in 1896 by studying uranium salts, and went on to research this newly discovered phenomenon alongside the Curies, eventually sharing the Nobel Prize in Physics with the couple in 1903. He died in Le Croisic (western France) in 1908.

Marie quickly developed the hypothesis that this radiation comes from the atom and that, if radium emits it, other elements must do so too. She began systematically studying all the elements that had been identified by that time, and observed that thorium emitted the same type of rays. She subsequently discovered a new element which emitted even greater levels of what she called "radioactivity", but although she could see it under the microscope, she was unable to isolate it to prove its existence.

Pierre Curie then abandoned all the projects he was working on to help his wife. Thanks to their perseverance, they eventually located this highly radioactive substance in a uranium-based mineral called pitchblende, and Marie named it polonium in homage to her native country. A few days later, the couple managed to isolate radium, which was even more radioactive. However, at this stage their discovery was only theoretical, and they still had to prove the existence of these new substances to the scientific world.

FROM A RUN-DOWN LABORATORY TO A PROFESSORSHIP AT THE SORBONNE

The Curies devoted every day to extracting radium, sometimes even working through the night. To begin with, they faced two major problems: finding enough of the mineral to work with (buying it would be too expensive) and finding a place to work. On Rue Lhomond, in the courtyard of the School of Physics, there was a dilapidated, disused hangar which had formerly served as a dissection room. The Curies were delighted when they were given permission to use it, in spite of its very rudimentary facilities. This was followed by a piece of good news from

Austria: the Austrian government was prepared to give them a tonne of pitchblende residue if they would pay for it to be transported to Paris.

Marie carried out much of the heavy work in the courtyard while Pierre worked with vials and test tubes. With her sleeves rolled up and her apron and hands badly damaged by the acid, she spent hours stirring the boiling material in a vast iron basin, surrounded by dense smoke, in order to extract pure radium salts. In 1902, four years after she had first announced the probable existence of the new element, she finally managed to prepare a decigram of it and made an initial calculation of its atomic mass. Her fellow scientists were still sceptical about radium's existence and believed that only an exact calculation of its atomic mass could prove that it really existed. Marie and Pierre's aim was therefore to extract a decigram of it in order to isolate the element and determine its exact properties. Their tireless work paid off, as they managed to prove beyond all doubt that radium existed.

On 25 June 1903, Marie was finally able to defend her thesis, and on 10 December of the same year, she shared the Nobel Prize in Physics with Pierre and Henri Becquerel. She was the first woman to be awarded a Nobel Prize in any discipline, and also became the first woman to receive the Davy Medal, which is awarded by the Royal Society of London "for an outstandingly important recent discovery in any branch of chemistry". On 10 December 1911, she received her second Nobel Prize, this time in chemistry, for her work on radium and polonium, making her the first person to receive the award twice.

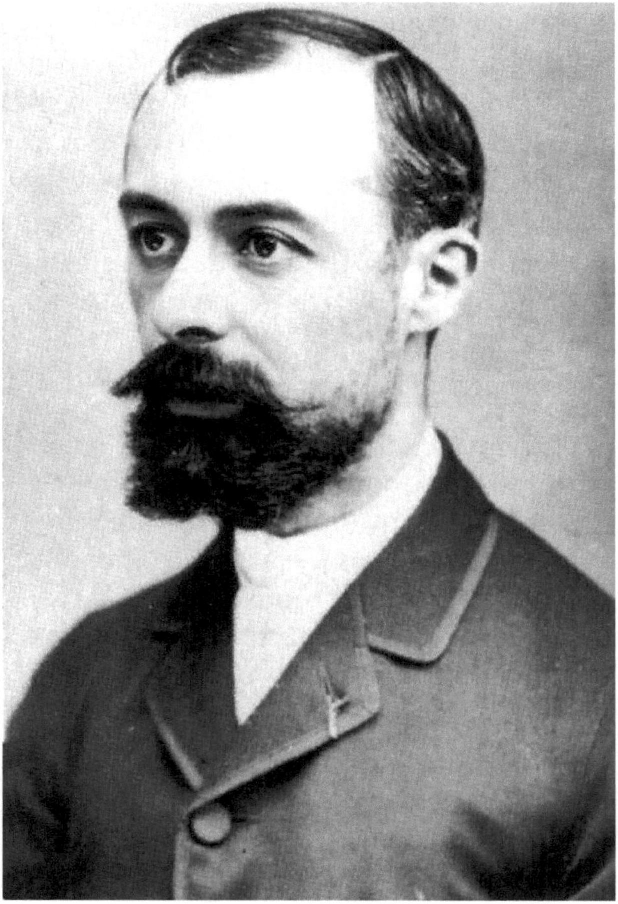

| Photograph of Henri Becquerel, 19th century.

In 1904, Marie gave birth to her second daughter, Ève (1904-2007). Two years later, Pierre died suddenly and unexpectedly in an accident involving a horse-drawn vehicle. His death hit Marie hard, but her commitment to her scientific career did not waver. That year, she took over the professorship left vacant by his death, and in doing so became the first woman to teach at the Sorbonne. She became a titular professor in 1908, and remained in the post until 1934.

Radioactivity in numbers

Polonium (Po), the first radioactive element discovered by the Curies, has the atomic number 84. Radium (Ra), which was discovered afterwards and has the atomic number 88, is one million times more radioactive than uranium and its most stable isotope has a half-life (the time taken for a substance to lose half its radioactivity) of 1600 years.

The atomic number refers to the number of protons in the nucleus of the atom of a given element. The element's properties are determined by this charge rather than by its mass.

THE RADIUM INSTITUTE AND THE SEARCH FOR A CANCER TREATMENT

Marie remembered that when Pierre had worked with radioactive substances, he had noticed that they affected his skin: while they sometimes gave him burns, they also helped certain wounds to heal. In tests on animals, the couple had observed that exposure to radiation caused cancerous tumours to shrink. However, they had opted not to patent the procedure, and instead made their work on the properties of radioactivity available to any interested researchers. They felt that profiting from their discoveries was contrary to the spirit of scientific endeavour, even though this would have provided them with the money they needed to finance the research laboratory they had long dreamed of.

In late 1909, Pierre Paul Émile Roux (1853-1933), a French professor and the director of the Pasteur Institute, suggested creating an institute dedicated to radium (which later became known as the Curie Institute) for the purpose of carrying out medical research into cancer and developing new treatments based on radiotherapy. The premises were completed in 1914, and Roux placed Curie and Claudius Regaud (French doctor and biologist, 1870-1940) in charge of the institute. The plan was for Regaud to study hybrid treatments combining X-rays and radiotherapy. During the First World War (1914-1918), the Institute temporarily suspended its activity, and Marie threw herself into treating the wounded, in particular by requisitioning cars to set up mobile radiography units, which played a crucial role in detecting bullets embedded in the men's bodies and evaluating the after-effects of their injuries.

In 1918, research resumed at the Radium Institute, and Marie's daughter Irène began working as her assistant. Numerous foreign students and physicists came from all over the world to learn about radiography. Many of these visitors were women, and Marie, who remembered how difficult it had been for her to access higher education because of her gender, welcomed them to her lab, which opened doors in the scientific world for them. In 1921, the American journalist Marie Meloney (1878-1943) collected $100 000 from women in the USA to purchase one gram of pure radium for the Institute. When Curie travelled to the USA to receive the radium from President Warren G. Harding (1865-1923), she was greeted with great enthusiasm. She met and became friends with the German-born physicist Albert Einstein (1879-1955), and worked alongside him as part of the International Committee on Intellectual Cooperation, an advisory organisation for the League of Nations (an intergovernmental organisation which was active from 1920 to 1946, before being superseded by the United Nations) which worked to coordinate scientific research and relations on an international level.

Curie had been exposed to high levels of radiation from radioactive elements since 1898, and in the early 1920s she began to suspect that this exposure was responsible for the myriad health problems she was suffering from (she underwent numerous eye and ear operations from 1923 onwards), but remained reluctant to publicly discuss the dangers associated with radioactivity. She subsequently developed leukaemia as a result of her constant contact with radioactive substances, and became increasingly weak. She moved into the Sancellemoz sanatorium in Passy, Haute-Savoie on 29 June 1934 and died there on 4 July after suffering from severe bouts of bronchitis and flu.

POLITICAL, SOCIAL AND ECONOMIC CONTEXT

WOMEN'S LACK OF ACCESS TO EDUCATION

Poland was occupied by Russia for the majority of the 19th century, starting in 1815 during the reign of Tsar Alexander I (1777-1825). In 1831, under the reign of Nicholas I (1796-1855), Poland lost its status as a sovereign state and became part of Congress Poland, which was created in 1815 by the Congress of Vienna. Poland remained under Russian control until 1915, when the territory was ceded to the invading German and Austrian forces.

One consequence of this state of affairs was that the education of Polish children was strictly controlled by the Russian authorities. Girls were hit particularly hard by these restrictions, as they were forbidden from attending university. This gave rise to underground student groups organised by Polish professors for young women, who had realised that their freedom depended on their access to education, as well as to young men from all social backgrounds. One such group was the Flying University, an illegal institution created in 1885 after a Polish rebellion was brutally repressed by the Russians, which Curie attended as a young woman. The Flying University provided education for thousands of men and women, including the novelist and dramatist Zofia Nałkowska (1884-1954) and the educator, author and pedagogue Janusz Korczak (1878-1942), between 1885 and 1905 in response to Russian domination.

The situation was not as dire in France, but the country's education system was still far from equal. Although women had been granted access to the universities in 1880, they remained a small minority in institutions of higher education and were a long way from being considered equal to men. In 1884, the French philosopher and scientist Clémence Royer (1830-1902) became the first woman to lecture at the Sorbonne, although the university refused to give her the title of professor. Similarly, Curie was not immediately recognised as a titular professor when she began teaching there.

INDUSTRIAL AND SCIENTIFIC PROGRESS DURING THE *BELLE ÉPOQUE*

The period between the end of the 19th century and the outbreak of the First World War in 1914 was characterised by unprecedented industrial development. Rapid scientific and technological progress gave rise to a number of major changes: transport was revolutionised first by the steam engine, then by electricity, and industrial production and communications systems developed faster than ever before.

Capitalism developed and soon became the dominant economic and political system in Western Europe, bringing with it major social changes as citizens migrated en masse from the countryside to the rapidly growing cities in the hope of finding work in the new factories. This in turn led to the emergence of the working class. At the same time, scientific and medical progress lowered the death rate, in particular the infant mortality rate.

At the dawn of the 20th century, research in the field of physics took a new direction: rather than focusing on phenomena that could be observed by the human eye, physicists turned their attention to the world of atoms and electrons, which enabled them to develop hypotheses about the universe and its structure and about astrophysics. There were two reasons for this shift:

- **Greater emphasis on scientific education.** Men such as the French philosopher Ernest Renan advocated more widespread scientific education and the study of the sciences as a subject in their own right (prior to this time, they were considered secondary to literary studies).
- **The Industrial Revolution in Europe during the 19th century.** This resulted in major progress in many fields of science and technology, including medicine and physics. During this period, researchers in every domain were chiefly concerned with progress, and it did not matter to them whether this progress was a result of conscious effort or came about by chance. This paved the way for the discoveries of Louis Pasteur (French chemist and biologist, 1822-1895) and, later, Albert Einstein.

The theories that had been accepted during the

19th century collapsed in a matter of decades, and were superseded by new scientific ideas and theories, including:

- Einstein's theories of special relativity and general relativity;
- Max Planck's (German physicist, 1858-1947) quantum theory, which sought to model the behaviour of energy on a small scale;
- the theory of uranium rays developed by Henri Becquerel;
- electrolysis (a method which uses electric currents to change the chemical composition of a substance), which became widely used to prepare metals;
- the development of the first plastic materials, such as Bakelite;
- Édouard Branly's (French physicist and doctor, 1844-1910) development of wireless telegraphy.

When the First World War broke out, the French government sought to further encourage scientific advances to help in the fight against Germany.

THE RISE OF FEMINISM

The early 20th century was also a period of progressive social development in France, as the growth of the working class gave rise to struggles for justice, equal rights and greater fairness in the world of work. The early French feminists drew inspiration from the activism and courage of their British counterparts, the suffragettes.

The feminist struggle in England

The suffragettes were the members of the Women's Social and Political Union, which was founded in England in 1903 and aimed to secure women's right to vote. In their bid to secure political equality, they resorted to direct action, which was often spectacular and attention-grabbing: for example, they interrupted public meetings to bring their demands to a wider audience and chained themselves to the railings outside Parliament. However, the movement was brutally repressed and its members were imprisoned, violently attacked or even killed. However, their efforts paid off in 1918, when married women over the age of 30 were finally granted the right to vote.

This was a period of relative political stability in France, which allowed citizens to focus their attention on progress rather than fearing further social disorder. Thanks to an early demographic boom, France was now the most populous country in Europe. Food supplies increased, medical advances reduced the mortality rate, and women gradually gained control over their own lives and were increasingly able to pursue their own careers.

In this promising context, Curie was able to pursue her research on Becquerel's uranium rays and garner recognition as a scientist.

KEY MOMENTS

HENRI BECQUEREL'S INFLUENCE

In 1896, Henri Becquerel had observed that certain minerals containing uranium emitted rays which shared some characteristics with the X-rays discovered by Wilhelm Röntgen. All that he was able to do was discover that these rays came from within the substance rather than being caused by external forces and identify some of their effects, such as the darkening of photographic plates or the ionisation of the air (this occurs when neutral atoms gain or lose electrons, turning them into charged ions, which means that the surrounding air becomes electrified) as indicated by an electroscope (a piece of equipment for measuring electric charge).

Marie's decision to study these rays was influenced by her husband Pierre's work: in 1880, he had discovered piezoelectricity, meaning an electric charge which appears on certain substances when mechanical stress is applied. Thanks to this discovery, he and his brother

Jacques were able to develop a system to measure very small electrical charges. Their device consisted of an ionisation chamber (a sort of particle detector which calculates the total charge of the electrons present in the ions) and a quadrant electrometer. It played a crucial role in the early days of measuring radioactivity, as very precise measurements of radiation would allow its origins to be identified. In this way, Pierre's device enabled Marie to advance very quickly in her research.

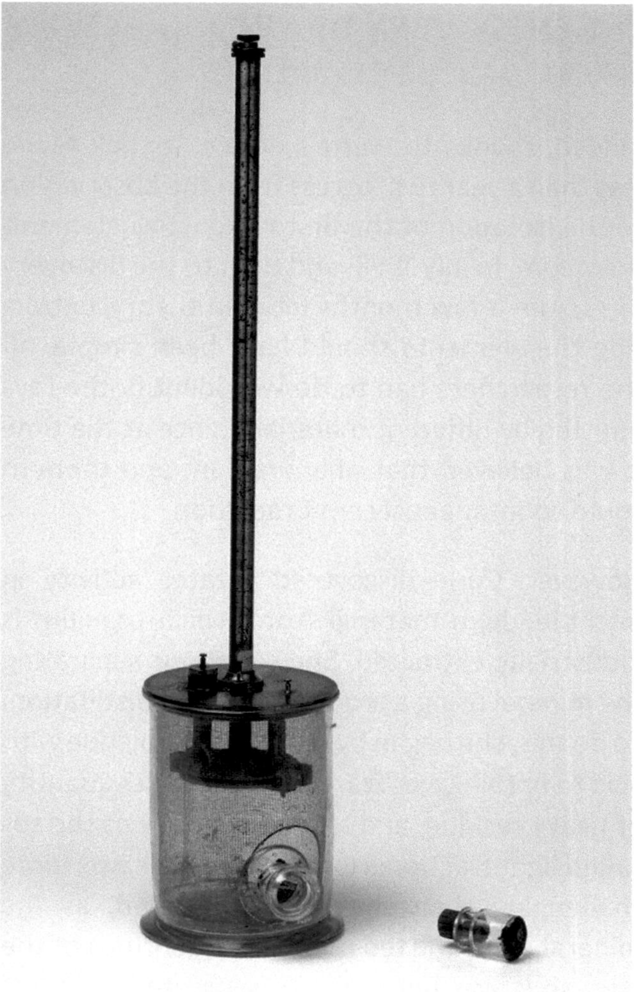

| Pierre Curie's quadrant electrometer.

THE DISCOVERY OF TWO RADIOACTIVE ELEMENTS

Indeed, thanks to Pierre's device, it took Marie less than a year to progress from the observation to the isolation of the first radioactive element, polonium, in July 1898, and then to the discovery of radium a few months later. In theory, extracting the elements should have been simple: all the researchers had to do was identify the rays emitted by different materials, since at the time it was believed that only uranium and thorium could spontaneously emit radiation.

However, Curie discovered greater activity in pitchblende, a material from which uranium is industrially extracted. She set about separating the mineral using a process similar to distillation. To do this, she began by heating pitchblende with acid to obtain two "fractions": a smaller quantity of heavy residue, and a large quantity of the so-called light fraction. However, the task was more challenging than she had anticipated, as the mineral only emitted miniscule quantities of the rays, so it was necessary to separate enormous quantities of the rock to observe them. It was slow, arduous work, but Curie pressed on and her experiments with pitchblende eventually led her to discover two new elements, namely radium, which came from the "heavy" residue, and polonium, which was found in the "light" distillate and was far more radioactive.

Calculating radium's atomic mass

After Curie successfully isolated radium in 1910, the next step was to determine its atomic mass. To do so, she prepared radium chloride, then added silver nitrate in order to precipitate the chloride ions. As she already knew the atomic masses of chlorine and silver, determining the mass of the precipitated silver chloride enabled her to deduce the mass of chlorine in the initial radium chloride, and then use simple subtraction to obtain radium's atomic mass.

RADIOACTIVITY AND THE CHALLENGING OF ESTABLISHED BELIEFS

The discovery of two new elements and of radioactivity sent shockwaves through the scientific community, as these discoveries profoundly challenged some of the major scientific theories that had prevailed since ancient Greece. Specifically, it had always been believed that matter was indivisible and eternal, and consequently that there were a fixed number of stable atoms in the universe, which was viewed as a fragmented space comprising vacuums and areas where there was matter. This meant that 19th-century scientists believed that chemical processes were the only things that could influence atomic activity. However, Curie demonstrated that the radiation she had observed had a physical, not a chemical, cause.

TWO NOBEL PRIZES

In November 1903, the Royal Society of London awarded Curie the prestigious Davy Medal, one of the greatest honours a scientist could receive.

As she was ill at the time, Pierre attended the ceremony on her behalf. One month later, on 10 December 1903, the Royal Swedish Academy of Sciences announced that that year's Nobel Prize in Physics would be jointly awarded to Henri Becquerel, Pierre Curie and Marie Curie for their discovery of and research into radioactivity. In addition to the honour that this represented, the award came with a 70 000-franc prize, which gave Pierre the opportunity to leave his teaching post at the School of Physics and devote himself to research full-time. He was replaced by the French philosopher of science and pedagogue Paul Langevin (1872-1946). The couple also hired an assistant, gave money to struggling acquaintances, including Polish students, laboratory workers and one of Marie's childhood friends, and made financial contributions to scientific societies.

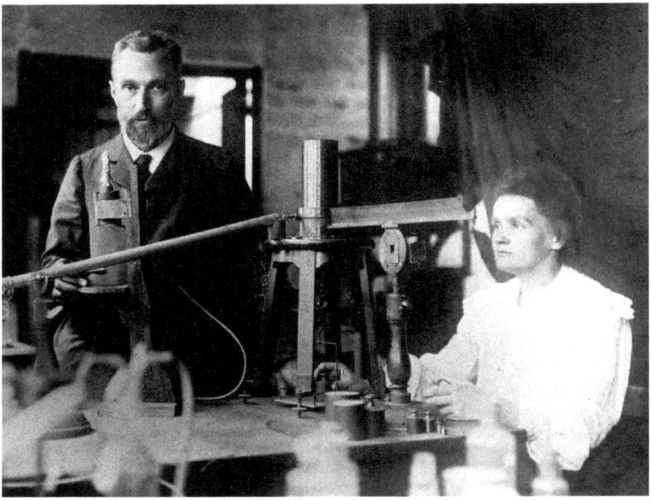

| Pierre and Marie Curie in their laboratory, c. 1904.

1911 was a big year in the scientific world. From 30 October to 3 November, the first of the Solvay Conferences (so called because they were organised by the Belgian chemist and industrialist Ernest Solvay [1838-1922]) was held in Brussels and attracted some of the biggest names in science, including Einstein and the French physicist Jean Perrin (1870-1942). The theme of the conference was *Radiation and Quanta*, and scientists had the opportunity to freely discuss current advances in the field and their work.

Curie was the only woman present, a state of affairs that was to persist for many years.

On 8 November of that year, after losing her husband and research partner, Curie was awarded the Nobel Prize in Chemistry "in recognition of her services to the advancement of chemistry by the discovery of the elements radium and polonium, by the isolation of radium and the study of the nature and compounds of this remarkable element".

However, this professional triumph was accompanied by personal heartache, as her alleged relationship with Paul Langevin (who was married but estranged from his wife) tarnished her reputation and led her to be labelled a "home-wrecker". The scandal surrounding the affair was exacerbated by the misogyny and xenophobia that characterised French society at the time. Although the Nobel Committee tried to dissuade her from travelling to Stockholm because of political pressure and the scale of the controversy, she was undeterred and went to collect the prize in person.

RADIOTHERAPY AND ITS IMPACT ON MEDICINE

Thanks to its novel properties, radium remained the object of increasing interest until the 1940s. It was used in various fields, including radiotherapy, pharmacology and industry, and even in everyday life.

In early 1900, the German researchers Otto Walkhoff (1860-1934) and Friedrich Giesel (1852-1927) identified radium's physiological properties. Pierre Curie was intrigued by their discovery, and decided to work with them to study these properties. In experiments on animals, he discovered that radium could be used to heal wounds and even eliminate tumours. In June 1901, Pierre Curie and Henri Becquerel published a paper on the physiological effects of radium rays, marking the beginning of radiotherapy.

These new techniques could be used to treat cancer, and the results of early investigations into their potential for treating a variety of skin conditions were encouraging. Medical professionals began to see radium as a promising option for a panoply of medical conditions for which no cure existed at the time, including tuberculosis. Enthusiasm for brachytherapy (a form of radiotherapy which involves temporarily inserting radioactive substances into the body next to the area to be treated), which was precise, effective and could be used in high concentrations, swept around the world. The Curies' work therefore marked a new frontier in medicine, as it provided doctors with a new weapon against cancer.

The use of radiation in medicine

Brachytherapy involves using needles or dressings to bring the radioactive substance into direct contact with the wound or tumour to be treated. The substance is placed in a sealed container and applied to or inserted directly into the area for treatment, for example in the cases of cervical cancer or prostate cancer. In radiotherapy, the patient remains at a distance from the rays, so the procedure tends to be slightly less effective, particularly if the person moves during treatment.

OTHER MEDICAL APPLICATIONS

Radium quickly proved to be a potent weapon in the fight against cancer and tumours, but this was not its only use: radiography was invaluable during the First World War, as it allowed bullets to be precisely located within wounded soldiers' bodies, making it easier to surgically remove them.

Curie threw herself into the war effort, notably by requisitioning cars belonging to civilians in order to set up mobile surgical units. This allowed 18 radiography units to be sent to the front. Although some soldiers had never heard of this new treatment and were worried that it was going to be painful, Curie reassured them by telling them that it was no different to having their photograph taken (Curie, 2001).

THE END OF RADIUM

Although the discovery of radium was undeniably a major step forward in the fight against cancer, it was not long before its negative effects became apparent. It is an exceptionally radioactive substance (it is a million times more radioactive than uranium) and can be very dangerous to humans, as was the case for the medical staff who handled it. As early as 1921, its harmful effects were already noticeable, and much stricter security measures were made compulsory: the walls of the rooms where radiotherapy was to be carried out had to be reinforced with lead, and a strict set of rules had to be followed when handling radium. However, these precautions were not enough to make the substance completely safe.

Before long, pure radium was abandoned in favour of safer radioactive substances. Marie and Pierre's daughter Irène Curie and her husband, the French physicist and chemist Frédéric Joliot (1900-1958) discovered artificial radioactivity in 1934, and in the same year illnesses resulting from the production of radium salts were officially recognised as occupational illnesses in France. In 1937, its use was banned outside the field of medicine. In 1976, it was abandoned in radiotherapy and replaced by iridium-192 and caesium-137, which are significantly less toxic.

IMPACT

IRÈNE AND FRÉDÉRIC JOLIOT-CURIE AND THE DISCOVERY OF ARTIFICIAL RADIOACTIVITY

Irène Curie worked alongside Marie for much of her life, and shared her mother's passion for physics, chemistry and medicine. At the end of the First World War in 1918, she became her mother's assistant at the Radium Institute. She was in charge of training engineers in nuclear chemistry, which was how she met her husband Frédéric Joliot. The couple had two children together: Hélène in 1927 and Pierre in 1932. Like Marie and Pierre Curie, they formed a close professional partnership, driven by their shared goal of discovering artificial radioactivity by transforming a stable element into a radioactive element. They succeeded in 1934, shortly before Marie's death, and were rewarded with the Nobel Prize in Chemistry the following year. Their achievement represented an important step towards nuclear fission (the splitting of the nucleus of an atom into multiple smaller nuclei, resulting in the release of thermal energy).

Irène Joliot-Curie became the director of the Radium Institute in 1946, and also headed the French Alternative Energies and Atomic Energy Commission and was appointed to the professorship previously held by her mother. She died in 1956 from leukaemia resulting from high levels of radiation exposure throughout her life.

THE CURIE FOUNDATION AND GROUNDBREAKING CANCER TREATMENTS

The Radium Institute, founded in 1909, was an important research and treatment hub which greatly facilitated the development of radiotherapy. Curie and Claudius Regaud's constant fundraising efforts culminated in the creation of the Curie Foundation in 1920. It was recognised as a public-interest institute the following year, and had two objectives: to finance the Radium Institute's activities, and to help develop its treatment units. In 1922, a dispensary was built on the Rue Ulm, and an anonymous donation in 1923 was used to build new biology laboratories.

When Irène Joliot-Curie received her Nobel Prize in 1935, cancer patients flocked to the Radium Institute, and before long a new building became necessary. Accordingly, the Curie hospital, which was run by the Institute, was opened in 1936 and expanded in 1956. In 1965, an eight-storey general hospital replaced the dispensary, and in 1970 the Radium Institute and the Curie Foundation merged into a single body, the Curie Institute, which focuses on research, teaching and cancer treatment. On 1 January 2010, in response to the increasing challenge posed by cancer, the Curie Institute merged with the Centre René Hugeunin to become one of Europe's leading oncology centres.

APPLICATIONS IN ISOTOPE GEOCHEMISTRY

Radium's impact extended beyond the field of medicine: the rays it emits allow luminescent paint which emits weak but continuous light to be produced using a mixture of radium salts and zinc sulphide. Paint containing radium became widespread in the early 20th century, notably in the mass-production of clocks with fluorescent faces and in the development of road markings and signs that would be visible at night.

However, aside from its medical applications, undoubtedly the greatest scientific advance resulting from the discovery of radiation was radiocarbon dating, which involves using radioactive isotopes (notably carbon-12 and carbon-14) to determine the age of objects such as human bones. Measuring the quantity of carbon that has been lost in relation to the substance's atomic mass allows scientists to calculate their age and identify the time period they date from.

THE DANGERS OF RADIATION

As radium became more widely used, its harmful effects became clear. In the USA, the female factory workers who painted luminescent clock hands later became known as "Radium Girls", and as well as using their tongue or teeth to point their brushes, they also sometimes painted their lips and nails with radium to surprise their boyfriends in the dark. They were unaware of the risks they were running until it was too late, as nobody had warned them about the dangers, even though their supervisors were careful to avoid too much exposure to the radioactive substances. Within just a few years, 43 Radium Girls had died, while others suffered from anaemia, bone fractures and necrosis of the jaw.

Radium Girls

The factory worker Grace Fryer (1899-1933) was the first Radium Girl to take legal action against her employer, as her colleagues were afraid that the scandal, which was covered extensively in the media, would harm their reputations. Once Fryer had taken the first steps, it took five more workers and two years to find a lawyer willing to represent them and get their case heard. The plaintiffs each received $10 000 in compensation, and new rules were implemented to protect workers and to give them the right to take legal action against their employers.

Furthermore, radium was initially seen as a way of ensuring a more youthful complexion, and cosmetics companies began producing ointments, compresses and drinkable solutions, including the famous cream *Tho-Radia*, which bore a label stating that it used Dr Alfred Curie's special formula. Although Alfred Curie was in no way connected to Marie and Pierre, attaching his name to the product reassured consumers and boosted sales. Radium was believed to be completely safe, and in 1916 the medical journal *Radium* assured readers that the element was not at all toxic and that the body accepted it naturally.

Radium was used to treat a whole host of illnesses, from heart problems to impotence to depression. It is difficult to calculate the total number of victims, but we can say with certainty that the presence of radium in everyday life was a contributing factor in many cases of leukaemia and other health problems, including physical deformities and intellectual disabilities in newborns, a rise in genetic illnesses and sarcomas.

A PIONEERING WOMAN

When her husband died and she took over his professorship at the Sorbonne, Curie became the first female professor there. Even more impressively, at 39 she was young to be stepping into such a prestigious teaching position. This, in combination with her two Nobel Prizes, cemented her reputation as a leading scientist and intellectual and made her a model to follow for subsequent generations of women. She spent her entire life breaking barriers, starting in her early years in Russian-occupied Poland when she defied the authorities by joining the clandestine Flying University. She refused to let the fact that women in Poland were barred from higher education hold her back; instead, she learnt French and left to study in Paris.

Although Curie had no shortage of detractors because of her gender, she never failed to confound their expectations and show other women that they did not need to rely on men to be successful. Her daughters followed her example: Irène won her own Nobel Prize in 1935, while Ève went on to become a brilliant writer and journalist. Her 1938 biography of her mother, *Madame Curie*, immediately shot to the top of the bestseller lists.

The Curies' years of tireless work resulted in a legacy that endured long after their deaths. In 1995, the French president François Mitterrand (1916-1996) expressly requested that their bodies be transferred from Seaux to the Panthéon, a mausoleum for France's most distinguished citizens, where they were buried side by side. Marie became the second woman to be buried there, after Sophie Berthelot (1837-1907), the wife of the scientist Marcellin Berthelot (1827-1907), and the first woman to be buried there on her own merits.

Curie's coffin was designed to protect her surroundings from the high radiation levels in her body, and comprised three layers: an outer layer of wood, an inner layer of lead and then another layer of wood. In 1995, experts measured the radiation emitted by her body and concluded that it had finally reached safe levels, but as a precautionary measure she is still buried in a lead-lined coffin.

SUMMARY

- Maria Salomea Skłodowska was born in Warsaw in 1867 to parents who shared a thirst for knowledge and a passion for physics and mathematics. She was a precocious child who could read perfectly by the age of four and took an early interest in mathematics. However, at this time Poland was governed by Russia, which meant that the school curriculum was tightly controlled and women were barred from attending university.
- As a young woman, she worked as a governess for a family of farm owners and secretly taught groups of Polish children.
- In 1891, she moved to Paris to join her sister, who was finishing her studies there. She enrolled at the Sorbonne and began calling herself Marie, the French version of Maria. Although she lived in abject poverty, she threw herself into her studies, at which she excelled. In 1894, she met her future husband, Pierre Curie, and the couple worked together on her research for her doctoral thesis on radioactivity, which

had been discovered but not fully explained by Henri Becquerel. The Curies and Becquerel were jointly awarded the Nobel Prize in Physics in 1903 for their groundbreaking work on the phenomenon.

- When Pierre was killed in a road accident in 1906, Marie took over his professorship at the Sorbonne, making her the first woman to serve as a professor at the university. Alongside her teaching, she continued her research on radium.
- In 1909, Curie and Claudius Regaud founded the Radium Institute, which focused on research into radium and cancer treatment.
- In 1910, she successfully isolated radium for the first time, and as a result was awarded a second Nobel Prize, this time in chemistry, the following year.
- During the First World War, she requisitioned cars with dynamos and photography equipment in order to set up mobile radiography units, which were used behind the lines to examine and treat wounded soldiers. After the end of the war, she returned to her work at the Radium Institute and hired her daughter Irène as an assistant.

- In 1920, she used money donated by American women to purchase her first gram of radium. When she travelled around the USA in 1921, she was met with widespread acclaim and enthusiasm. However, her exposure to radium from 1898 onwards had begun to take its toll: she was left weakened by illness and returned to France in a state of profound exhaustion.
- She continued to teach at the Sorbonne to the best of her ability and to advocate on behalf of the Radium Institute. However, in 1934 she was admitted to the Sancellemoz sanatorium in Passy, Haute-Savoie suffering from radiation-induced leukaemia. She died in June of that year, but her daughter Irène Joliot-Curie continued her work and was rewarded with her own Nobel Prize in 1935.

We want to hear from you!
Leave a comment on your online library
and share your favourite books on social media!

FIND OUT MORE

BIBLIOGRAPHY

- Curie, È. (2001) *Madame Curie: A Biography.* Cambridge, Massachussetts: Da Capo Press.
- Frilley, M. (2004) Curie (les). *Encyclopédie Universalis*. Vol. 17. Paris: Encyclopaedia Universalis. pp. 1022-1028.
- Henry, N. (2015) *Les sœurs savantes, Marie Curie et Bronia Dluska*. Paris: Vuibert.
- Himbert, M-N. (2014) *Marie Curie, Portrait d'une femme engagée*. Paris: Actes Sud.
- Lejeune, D. (2003) *La France de la Belle Époque, 1896-1914*. Paris: Armand Colin.
- (2003) *Le Petit Larousse illustré*. Paris: Larousse.
- (No date) Marie Curie Physique et chimie – 1903/1911. *UPMC*. [Online]. [Accessed 8 March 2018]. Available from: <http://www.upmc.fr/fr/universite/histoire_et_personnalites/les_prix_nobel/marie_curie_physique_et_chimie_1903_1911.html>
- Montellier, C. (2011) *Marie Curie, la fée du radium.* Charleroi: Dupuis.
- Radvanyi, P. (2005) *Les Curie, pionniers de l'atome.* Paris : Belin.

- Savigneau, J. (2015) La révolution des suffragettes. *Le Monde*. [Online]. [Accessed 8 March 2018]. Available from: <http://www.lemonde.fr/televisions-radio/article/2015/11/26/la-revolution-des-suffragettes_4817529_1655027.html>

ADDITIONAL SOURCES

- Bailey Ogilvie, M. (2010) *Marie Curie: A Biography*. Westport: Greenwood Press.
- Emling, S. (2013) *Marie Curie and Her Daughters: The Private Lives of Science's First Family*. Basingstoke: Palgrave Macmillan.
- Moore, C. (2016) *The Radium Girls: The Dark Story of America's Shining Women*. London: Simon & Schuster.

ICONOGRAPHIC SOURCES

- Photograph of Marie Curie, c. 1903. Royalty-free reproduction picture.
- Photograph of Pierre and Marie Curie, 1903. Royalty-free reproduction picture.
- Photograph of Henri Becquerel, 19th century. Royalty-free reproduction picture.
- Pierre Curie's quadrant electrometer. © Science Museum London/Science and Society Picture Library.

- Pierre and Marie Curie in their laboratory, c. 1904. Royalty-free reproduction picture.

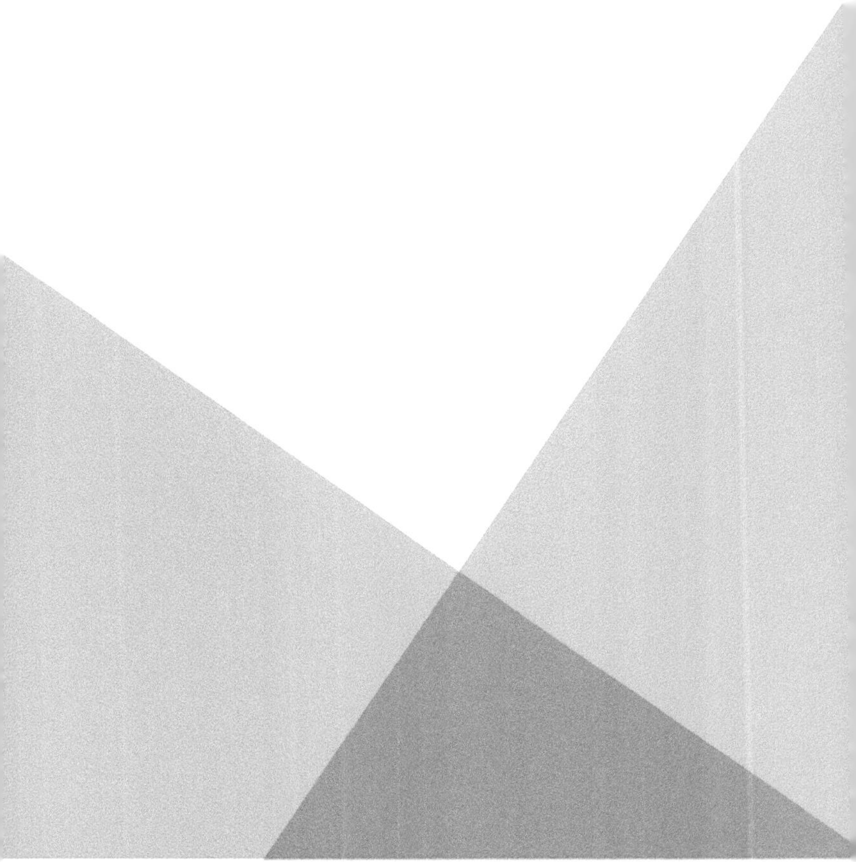

www.50minutes.com

Ebook EAN: 9782808008839

Paperback EAN: 9782808008846

Legal Deposit: D/2018/12603/196

Cover: © Primento

Digital conception by Primento, the digital partner of publishers.